RESTORING THE PELVIC FLOOR:

How Kegel Exercises, Vaginal Training, And Relaxation Solve Incontinence, Constipation, And Heal Pelvic Pain To Avoid Surgery

Dr. Amanda Olson, DPT, PRPC

Copyright 2018 Dr. Amanda Olson

Photos courtesy of Michaela Begg.

Dedicated to you dear reader.

*The knowledge and experience
I have gained is a gift to me,
but never mine to keep.*

Contents

Chapter 1

Introduction to the Pelvic Floor, Organs, Kegels and Women's Health

The pelvic floor and its associated issues have gained popularity in the past few years. Thanks to a growing number of resources, educational materials, outspoken women talking about their problems, and specialists treating these issues, more women are learning they are not alone in their struggles and that solutions may be available to them.

As a pelvic health physical therapist, I can't attend a baby shower, birthday party, wedding or meeting of any sort without someone cornering me and saying, "Hey, I need to ask you something privately."

My social media channels receive messages constantly from friends and strangers alike who ask questions about how to fix the women's issues that plague them. The fact that so many women have questions, combined with my strong notion that I'm a funny and convincing writer, but I'll let you be the judge, were the reasons for this book.

The Pelvis and the Pelvic Floor

A quick anatomy lesson will help you understand the concepts we will cover in this book. The pelvic girdle is composed of two crescent-shaped pelvic bones. These bones join at the front to form the pubic symphysis. They also join at the back on the triangle-shaped sacrum to form the sacroiliac joints.

The coccyx, or tailbone, attaches to the base of the sacrum. Finally, ligaments secure each of the joints, which connect bone to bone.

The pelvic floor muscles are a group of three distinct layers of muscles at the base of the pelvic girdle. They are not flat like the floor of a room is, though. At rest, they are domed downward. However, they are mobile and capable of squeezing inward and lifting upward in the pelvic cavity. The pelvic floor muscles consist of several muscles collectively.

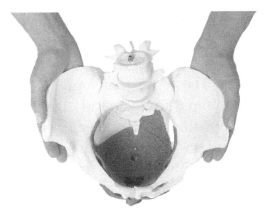

Top view of the pelvic floor muscles

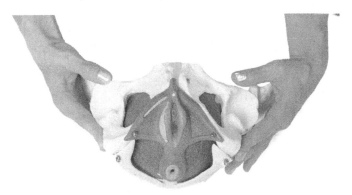

Bottom view of the pelvic floor. From top to bottom, passage of the urethra, vagina, and rectum are the three holes passing through the pelvic floor

However, for simplification and categorization, they are often referred to as the superficial urogenital muscles and the levator ani muscles. These muscles support the pelvic organs, rectum, uterus and bladder. The terminal openings of these organs pass through, and in females result in the three sphincteric openings of the anus, vagina and urethra.

Interestingly, men have a pelvic floor, too, which is similar in nature with the two terminal openings of the anus and urethra. Men suffer from pelvic floor dysfunctions as well, but this book will focus exclusively on issues pertaining to the female pelvic floor and female organs.

The following chapters will cover pelvic floor dysfunction and the related female issues of various natures. Some forms of pelvic floor dysfunction are due to a weakness or low tone of the pelvic floor. These issues commonly include urinary incontinence, pelvic organ prolapse, and in some cases, pelvic girdle pain.

In general, chronic pelvic pain in the absence of disease is because of muscles that are too tight. They require relaxation training, stretching, and most likely manual therapy from a trained pelvic floor physical therapist. There are also instances where women clench their pelvic floor muscles chronically. As a result, their pelvic floor muscles become shortened and lose flexibility, which can also result in urinary issues.

If you leak urine and also find yourself clenching your bottom during times of stress and or when you are lying in bed, this could be you. In such a case, you will want to review the chapters on relaxation and stretching of the pelvic floor muscles. Once you resolve these tendencies, you can then work on strengthening the muscles.

What I Do

As a pelvic health physical therapist, I treat a myriad of diagnoses including, but not limited to the following:

- Urinary incontinence and urinary urgency
- Mixed incontinence and fecal incontinence
- Constipation

- Pelvic and pubic pain
- Scar tissue and adhesions in the abdomen
- Post-Surgical Pain in the Abdomen and Pelvis
- Dyspareunia or pain during sex
- Vaginismus (pain during sex)
- Coccydynia (tailbone pain)
- Sacroiliac joint dysfunction
- Pregnancy-related pelvic girdle pain
- Pelvic floor dysfunction
- Post-prostatectomy pelvic floor dysfunction

Many people are unaware and shocked to learn that physical therapists specialize in these disorders. It takes several years of additional training to treat these issues effectively, and I have done my share. I have a doctorate degree in physical therapy and additional certification as a pelvic health rehabilitation specialist. Physical therapists have been treating these issues successfully for about 40 years, and it is becoming a more well-known specialty of health care.

Treatment of these issues requires a thorough review of the patient's medical history and an internal vaginal or rectal examination, depending on what the symptoms and issues are. Usually about midway through a vaginal examination a new patient will ask me, "So, what made you decide to go into this field?" I share my story because it is my why; why I do this, why I initially started training in this field, why I am passionate about what I do, and why I continue to absorb and learn all that I can about abdominal and pelvic health.

The story of how I became a pelvic physical therapist begins when I was in my mid-20s. I had completed my doctorate degree and was working in a children's hospital as a physical therapist specializing in pediatric neurology. I loved treating children and working in a collaborative research setting. One weekend, I found myself out on a camping trip where all the men were jumping off a rock into the river 40 feet below.

They scouted the area and determined it to be a safe place to land. Recap: I had a doctorate degree, so I was smart enough to know better and I was in my mid-20s, so I was old enough to know better.

Because I had a strong urge to keep up with boys, I jumped too. I landed in the seated position from a 40-foot drop. I am lucky that I did not damage my spinal cord and become paralyzed. However, I sustained a dislocation to my coccyx and significant damage to the muscles, tendons and ligaments of the pelvic floor. My husband had to fish me out of the river like a bug out of a pool and I couldn't sit for several months.

I went to a pelvic physical therapist who helped completely cure me of the pain and damage I had sustained. I healed without further issues after about six months of therapy. I even went on to have two baby boys naturally and without any issues during the delivery. At the end of my treatment, my pelvic physical therapist said to me, "Amanda, you need to quit pediatrics and do pelvic health. You have the right personality for it, and there is a huge need for more pelvic physical therapists."

One year later, I quit my job in pediatrics and went through the training process for credentialing as a pelvic physical therapist. This is absolutely my calling, and I love it. I can also say with the honest truth, when we are talking about pelvic floor dysfunction, that I may not be in your shoes, and I may not know exactly what you are going through, but I can appreciate how devastating these issues can be.

Pelvic pain hurts like nothing else I have experienced, and I have broken a leg and given birth naturally twice. This is not to minimize other issues, such as urinary incontinence or constipation. All pelvic floor issues are frustrating to some degree, but they are all "fixable."

What You Can Look Forward to Next

I firmly believe that Mary Poppins had it right: "A spoon full of sugar helps the medicine go down." I am not going to provide you with traditional medications, but with exercise and behavioral modifications to help you achieve your goals. In my professional practice and in life, I use humor as that spoon full of sugar to

It won't happen overnight, but a few key exercises and modifications will keep you dry, no matter what the circumstance.

Why Does Bladder Leakage Happen?

A little anatomy lesson can be helpful to understand how your plumbing works and why it can leak. The bladder is the holding vessel for urine, but it doesn't act up and start leaking without a reason. The bladder gets its support from a sling of muscles collectively called the pelvic floor muscles, as discussed in Chapter 1. There are three distinct layers of muscles: a superficial layer, a deep layer, and a layer of intermediary muscle and connective tissue in-between to hold these layers together.

These muscles form a diamond-shaped support sling, where the front anchors to the pubic bone, the back to the tailbone or coccyx, and the two sides to the ischial tuberosities, which are the bones you sit on. These muscles support the bladder, uterus and rectum. Each of these organs opens through the passages of the pelvic floor by way of the urethra where urine comes out, as well as the vagina and rectum, which leads to the anus.

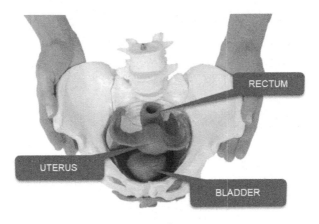

This image demonstrates the anatomy of the pelvic organs looking down into the pelvic bowl

Keep in mind that the bladder, uterus and rectum all live in the bony structure of the pelvis, so they are neighbors in tight quarters. They are essentially like campers in a tent that share nothing but a tent wall. Their neighbors that live directly above them are the intestines, liver, spleen and gallbladder.

They are all happy tenants of the abdomen and thorax condominium suites. The ceiling to this establishment is the diaphragm, which is the muscle in charge of drawing air in and out of your lungs. As you can see, this is a powerful section of the body that is busy carrying out important functions such as breathing, digestion and procreation, among other valuable tasks.

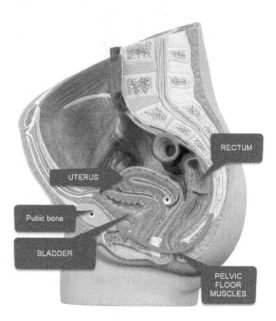

This image of a side view of the thorax with organs and pelvic floor muscles

The simple answer why bladder leakage occurs during forceful events such as coughing, sneezing and laughing is because the pressure above the bladder is greater than the pressure below it. For example, a sneeze comes on rapidly and causes a big squeeze in the abdomen as you expel whatever was tickling your nose. If your pelvic floor muscles don't respond by providing a tight, sturdy closure around the base of the bladder, all that force will crash down onto the bladder, and with nothing stopping it, urine will leak out.

Stress Urinary Incontinence

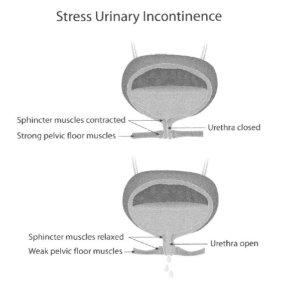

This image demonstrates the role of the pelvic floor muscles in providing closure around the urethra of the bladder.

Leakage: Understanding the Common Culprits

Yes, your muscles could be weak, but there could be other causes, too. Pregnancy and obesity can cause the pelvic floor muscles to stretch due to the increased weight above them, which can weaken them. Vaginal delivery of a baby can lead to tearing of the muscles, as well. High-impact sports and physical activity can also lead to pressure on the pelvic floor, which can weaken it with time.

A few common culprits include long-distance running, weightlifting, gymnastics, basketball, and track and field. Jobs that require heavy lifting or pushing can also lead to pressure on the pelvic floor that, over time, can lead to weakening. The great news is that just like any other muscle group, you re-strengthen and retrain them. Timing and coordination of the pelvic floor muscles can also be a factor in bladder leakage.

These muscles, just like other muscle groups, need to operate smoothly, synchronously and according to the fast instructions coming from the brain. When the organs and pelvic floor operate like a well-oiled machine, the muscles contract powerfully and lightning fast at the first sign of pressure from a cough, sneeze, laugh or jump. Events such as surgery to the abdomen or pelvis, delivery of a baby or chronic constipation can disrupt this smooth operation.

Surgery, no matter how small the scope was or how minimally invasive, can cause a mild disruption to the organs in the pelvis and the pelvic floor itself. The muscles can experience mild to moderate swelling, and during this time they can forget how to contract on time. Chronic constipation causes the pressure of a full rectum to compress the nerves and blood vessels of the pelvic floor muscles, which can also disrupt their timing. Don't worry, this is fixable.

There are also instances where the pelvic floor muscles are not weak. Instead, they are strong, yet too stiff. Some women and men have pelvic floor muscles that are too tight. If you can imagine Arnold Schwarzenegger trying to do yoga, you may understand how overly strong muscles can lose flexibility over time. This inflexibility can lead to poor coordination and the inability to contract on time to prevent leakage during a cough or sneeze.

So, if you are experiencing pelvic pain, pain during sex, or notice your hips and low back seem inflexible, you may also have tight pelvic floor muscles. A well trained pelvic physical therapist can help identify this and then create a program to improve the flexibility of your muscles to stop the leaking. Weakness and incoordination are two reasons why the pelvic floor may be supplying lower pressure during a sneeze. Many other factors can lead to the pressure being higher than normal above your bladder.

The most common of these is holding your breath during forceful activities. This includes exercise, or lifting a toddler or other heavy item. As discussed earlier, the diaphragm is the ceiling in the condominium analogy. When you hold your breath, the diaphragm presses downward into your abdomen. It then compresses the weight of all the other tenants (organs) downward as well, right over the top of the bladder.

If breath holding is a habit for you, it could lead to constant pressure over the top of your bladder. The pelvic floor has the responsibility of holding all this pressure, so over time, it can become tired. Thus, that strong hold around the base of the bladder can loosen, and then urine can escape.

Scar tissue in the abdomen can also cause the pressure to be greater above the bladder than it is below the pelvic floor, which can lead to leakage. Scar tissue from an appendectomy, hysterectomy, C-section, or other procedure on the stomach can even grow and stick to the bladder. The scar tissue is much thicker than the regular tissue in and around your organs. Little fingers of scar tissue can stick to its surrounding neighbors. When you bend over, twist or move about, your organs gently glide against each other. This allows you to be nimble and mobile. However, scar tissue can limit this motion, particularly in the event of a sneeze.

An excellent way to determine if you have a C-section scar that is too tight is to arch your back while standing. While arching your back, you may feel a pulling sensation in your skin or times. Do this exercise seven to eight times every day.

- You can verify that you are contracting the proper muscles by inserting one finger into your vagina and performing the Kegel. You should feel the muscles close all the way around the finger and draw it inward.

This action properly tightens the pelvic floor muscles around the urethra, and this is called a Kegel. Breathing is highly important during this exercise. Holding your breath will place pressure on the bladder and pelvic floor, thus making it difficult to contract your muscles properly. The breathing pattern for this exercise is to inhale and remain relaxed, then exhale as if you were cooling down hot food.

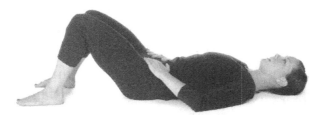

Research suggests that 80 Kegels per day are necessary to strengthen the pelvic floor and to keep women dry. Women who only do a few Kegels per day won't see an improvement in their bladder leakage. Remember, to successfully treat urinary incontinence, you must challenge your pelvic floor muscles so they become stronger.

If the steps above don't work for you, imagine that you are trying to shut off the flow of your urine. Practice this only once by urinating into the toilet and then stopping the flow of urine. This is referred to as the "stop test." Make sure you only perform it once or heavier weights to allow for gentle, incremental challenges to your pelvic floor muscles.

Here's how to find the proper weight to start your exercises:

- Place the lightest weight into your vagina just as you would a tampon.

- Stand up and attempt to hold the weight inside your vagina for one minute.

- If you can do that easily, try to walk around and do light household chores as you normally would with your clothing on, and while holding the weight inside for 10 to 15 minutes.

- When you achieve that step effortlessly, try the next heaviest weight on the following day.

- If the weight falls out into your underwear, go back down to the previous weight you were able to maintain for 15 minutes. Your pelvic floor muscles have to be actively engaged to keep the weight in and up.

- You can also place the weight in to perform the Kegel exercises. Because resistance is involved, you need far fewer Kegels to get the desired results.

- Make these exercises even more difficult by adding lubricant to the weight before you insert it. Using a lubricant makes the weight slippery and more challenging to hold inside your body.

- You can also gently pull on the string at the end of the weight. Pulling on the weight creates an eccentric muscle contraction because your muscles contract while lengthening. This form of exercise is highly beneficial in strengthening any muscle and can produce even faster results.

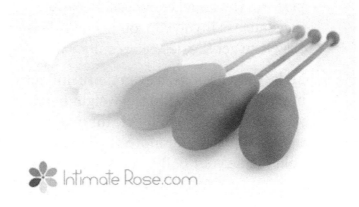

Look for advanced Kegel and Core Exercises in Chapter 6.

Chapter 3

Urinary Frequency and Urgency: Why Do I Have to Pee Every Time I Turn Around?

The need to urinate frequently is known as urinary frequency. It is often the companion of urinary urgency, which is the sudden urge to urinate with or without accidental urine leakage. Leakage may happen during certain activities, such as placing your key in your lock at home, while walking to the bathroom, or when you hear running water. It is fascinating to note that these are common everyday activities that afflict women consistently.

So, what does this say about the bladder? It is a sign that urinary frequency is mainly behavioral. That is, it has a "mind over matter" component to it. Bladder leakage that accompanies these urges is a real physiological phenomenon. The good news is, the brain is trainable and can turn this behavior around in time.

What Is Normal Bladder Behavior?

Normal bladder function is dependent on normal fluid consumption. Normal is often a gray area at best. We will discuss the role of diet and fluid consumption in Chapter 4. For now, the American Medical Association (AMA) and Mayo Clinic[1] recommend you drink when you are thirsty and according to your natural impulses.

However, most health experts previously recommended you drink approximately eight glasses of water per day. While this is probably still a good goal, researchers have not been able to determine what the optimal levels are. This is most likely because people come in different shapes and sizes. Also, they have different body temperatures and activity levels. These factors make it nearly impossible to make a blanket recommendation for all people regarding water.

The cells that make up our bodies are approximately 70 percent water. This means your daily intake of water is important to ensure these cells do their duties diligently. For example, increasing your physical activity or the exposure to hot temperatures will result in the loss of fluid via sweat. You will become thirsty and drink a little more under these conditions.

The female bladder can hold approximately 400 to 600 milliliters of fluid or eight to 12 ounces. Therefore, it is normal to urinate and empty that bladder every two to three hours. That makes for a grand total of eight trips to the bathroom per day. It is also typical to urinate a little during bowel movements. It is always a good idea to urinate before and after sex, so you get a few bonus rounds during such circumstances.

The average female should be able to sleep through the night without waking up to urinate until the age of 65, when it is natural to get up once per night. This is largely due to hormonal changes. If you are younger than 65 and waking up to urinate more than one or two times per night, take a close look at your fluid intake close to bedtime. If you are drinking two glasses of tea right before bed, then your bladder is going to be full and begging you to empty it.

You may consider withholding fluids after 7 p.m., or within approximately two to three hours before bedtime. If you are not drinking a lot of fluid before bedtime and still wake up frequently to urinate, bring this issue up with your health care provider. A few blood tests can help get to the bottom of your urinary frequency at night.

How to Train Your Brain to Control Your Bladder

Urinary frequency and urgency during the day are commonly due to certain habits, as we discussed, above. The most important factor in overcoming this form of incontinence is training your mind to maintain control over your bladder. One of the most common behaviors that lead to urinary frequency is going to the bathroom "just in case." As two-year-olds, your parents probably potty trained you under the pretense that you must always go to the restroom "just in case."

And for some people, this training persists over the years, leading to the bladder becoming confused as to what "full" truly means. For example, if you constantly empty your bladder in the morning before you leave for work, when you arrive at work and before leaving work when it's only half full at four ounces, the stretch receptors in the walls of your bladder become sensitized. You are training your bladder always to want to be empty it at that level.

Your bladder walls become sensitive to stretching beyond the halfway point. Once they reach the halfway point, they say, "Hey, lady, we are at four ounces here. That is usually when you empty me out. Please proceed to the restroom." And if you have the audacity to wait a few minutes, you might find that the urge goes away for a time before returning.

Have you ever had the experience where you had to use the restroom, but one was not readily available and then you forgot about it for another 45 minutes? This is your brain's ability to recognize that the first urgency warning was not a true alarm, but a first warning or suggestion.

Bladder urgency signals travel from the bladder through the spinal cord to the brain. They often come in two waves. The first one indicates the bladder is filling up. The second one indicates that "Now is the time to proceed to the restroom. Please and thank you."

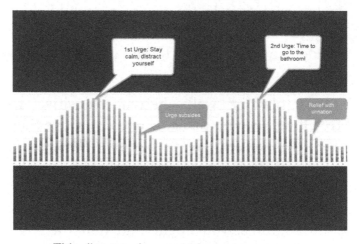

This diagram demonstrates urgency waves

What You Can Do About Your Bladder's Sudden Warning Signals

Sometimes the bladder's first warning can bring feelings of nervousness. This is because the bladder receives nerve input from the "fight-or-flight" system of nerves or the sympathetic nervous system. It also gets a signal from the "rest and restore" or the parasympathetic system. It is common for people to feel so scared, they pee their pants. In fact, this is a common saying.

But the reverse can also be true. Some women feel the urge to urinate and then it sends them into a fight-or-flight response. Their heart rate goes up, they begin scanning the room in search of the nearest restroom, and they walk as swiftly as possible in that direction. This response often leads to bladder leakage.

There is an adage in the pelvic health world that says, "If you get into a foot race with your bladder, it will win." So, it is important to walk calmly and normally. The most effective tool to counteract this fight-or-flight response is to tell yourself that you are in control of the situation and breathe calmly. Although it sounds bizarre, you must breathe slowly as you say these words in your head. These actions invoke higher brain control and will prevent your body from entering a fight-or-flight reaction.

Think of urgency as a wave, similar to an oceanic wave. There is a peak moment of heightened urgency. However, if you can remain calm and tell yourself you are in control, that wave of urgency will pass. After breathing deeply, perform two quick Kegels. The muscle contraction the pelvic floor muscles produce will send a signal to your bladder to momentarily relax.

This inhibits the strong sense of urgency due to the nerve connection between the spinal cord, the pelvic floor and the bladder. After the breathing, self-talk, and two quick Kegels, calmly proceed to a restroom.

Another method of stunting the strong urge to urinate is to sit down and place pressure on the perineum, or the area of muscles and tissues around the vagina. This is a method of bladder inhibition to prevent loss of urine during those moments of urgency. If you are in public and are not in the mood to grab your private parts in front of your work associates or friends, another party trick to prevent urine loss is to perform two quick pelvic floor contractions at the initial onset of the urgency.

This helpful technique inhibits the bladder from spasming or contracting and essentially tells it to calm down. You can perform them as many times as necessary before and while you calmly proceed to a toilet. The most critical component of Kegel exercises is that in addition to squeezing your pelvic floor muscles together, you draw the pelvic floor up simultaneously.

Be Patient: Time and Practice are the Keys to Bladder Control

These techniques are helpful when you find that your bladder isn't full each time you urinate. With time and practice, you will notice that you can delay your trips to the bathroom. Initially, you can help yourself by staying calm and distracting yourself. Look up a funny YouTube video on cats doing cute things, text a friend, stare out the window at something beautiful in nature - whatever strikes your fancy.

The goal is to gradually start spacing out bathroom trips by delaying by five minutes, then 10, then 20, and so on. After you delay going to the bathroom, the urge to go may dissipate and then return a second time. This signal is a strong indicator that you really do need to empty your bladder, so you should proceed to the restroom.

If delaying going to the bathroom doesn't diminish your urge and you know it's not bladder irritants as we will discuss in Chapter 4 discuss this matter with your health care provider. A provider can do an examination to determine how the muscles of your bladder are behaving. Then they can guide a more tailored approach to your bladder urges.

Another technique is known as "timed voiding." This method is beneficial for people who experience the urge to urinate followed soon by leaking urine. Oftentimes in this scenario, the bladder is not sending the signal to urinate until it is too full. Timed voiding is done by setting yourself on a schedule of going to the bathroom and urinating even if you don't feel the urge. You can set an alarm on your phone or watch at regular intervals, usually hourly or every 90 minutes, to remind you that it's time to go. You can begin to make these periods longer as your body adjusts and is able to make it the bathroom without having an accident.

Additionally, pelvic floor strengthening exercises, also referred to as Kegels, are beneficial in preventing urine leakage during times of urgency. We discussed these in Chapter 2.

The final consideration regarding bladder urgency and frequency is the consumption of bladder irritants in food and beverages. You're probably going to curse my name because it's all the fun things in life. If you keep them in check, you can still have your cake and hold your urine, too.

Diana's Story: Mind Over Matter

I had the pleasure of treating Diana for a few different diagnoses pertaining to the pelvic floor. She initially came to me because she was experiencing pelvic pain. During the course of treatment, Diane received the diagnosis of a genetic neurological disease. She began experiencing urinary urgency where she would feel a sudden and strong urge to urinate.

She often leaked once she crossed the threshold of the bathroom on the way to the toilet. I explained to her the role of the brain in overriding the fight-or-flight response. Although she laughed at the notion of talking to herself, thankfully, at that point she had grown to trust me and told me she would try it.

Diane's next appointment was just one week later. She was ecstatic to tell me how she had completely cured her urinary leakage with urgency by self-talk, deep breathing, two quick Kegels and staying calm. Diane was so elated with this response, she pondered the role of self-talk in other anxiety-provoking scenarios.

As a counselor, she began to use the notion of telling oneself, "I am in control. This is not an emergency, and everything will be okay," to help her clients overcome sensations of anxiety throughout their day. Diana's immediate success with stopping leakage during urinary urgency episodes is quite common. Once you experience the powerful notion that this form of urinary incontinence is simply mind over matter, you can create a new pattern of behavior and your leakage will stop.

Chapter 4

Bladder Irritants: Why What You Eat and Drink Can Be Irritating

Have you ever noticed the correlation between that extra cup of coffee and your occupation of the bathroom at work? Or have you heard that if you drink a lot of alcohol and have to go to the bathroom, you have "broken the seal"? But, there is no seal - only a bladder, bladder neck and pelvic floor. In fact, the reason behind your frequent trips to the bathroom is that your bladder is irritated, mad at you, and wants whatever you put in it to "get out."

Many women with bladder control problems limit their intake of liquids in hopes they will need to urinate less frequently or have less urinary leakage. While a reduction in liquid intake does result in a decrease in the volume of urine, the smaller amount of urine may be more highly concentrated. This highly concentrated urine will be dark yellow.

Interestingly, that dark, concentrated urine is more irritating to the inside of the bladder surface. It will cause you to go to the bathroom more frequently. Concentrated urine also encourages the growth of bacteria. More bacteria may lead to infections, resulting in incontinence.

The Common Urinary Culprits: Bladder Irritants

Bladder irritants are the chemicals you find in food and drinks. When you consume them, they encourage your bladder to send out the signal to urinate. These chemicals get filtered through the kidneys via your bloodstream. However, in higher doses, they settle into the walls of your bladder as it fills with urine. The best way to clear them out is by drinking water, maintaining hydration and urinating.

Everyone has different tolerance to these chemicals. A person with interstitial cystitis, a condition involving bladder pain and ulcers requiring a scope procedure to diagnose, knows that even small amounts of these chemicals can lead to exquisite pain and urinary frequency every 15 minutes. However, another person may get away with much higher amounts before noticing a slight uptick in their urge to urinate.

The foods and drinks most commonly associated with bladder irritation include[1]:

- All types of alcohol
- All kinds of caffeinated beverages
- Carbonated drinks
- Spicy foods
- Sugar and artificial sweeteners
- Chocolate
- Citrus fruits and other fruits:
  - Apples
  - Cantaloupe and pineapple
  - Grapes and plums
  - Cranberries and strawberries
  - Guava
  - Peaches
- Milk products like cheese, yogurt and ice cream

- Tomato-based products

- Vitamin B complex

- Vinegar

There are many items on this inclusive list that may or may not irritate your bladder. Pulling all of them out for a week or two and documenting your trips to the restroom is one way to determine your baseline. You can then gradually reintroduce items and keep documenting urinary frequency to help determine what irritates your bladder the most. Keeping a diary of the foods and drinks you consume, and your symptoms is also a great way to determine what gives you the most grief.

Your Bladder's Enemies: Irritants You Should Dump Now

It is important to note some items are going to irritate everybody's bladder. These include alcohol, caffeine, citrus and artificial sweeteners. It is often difficult and painful for long-time coffee drinkers to give up coffee entirely, especially all at once. You can decrease your daily intake as quickly as possible. However, a true dependence on caffeine can result in headaches and other physical and emotional discomfort.

Decrease at a rate that feels right for you. Some people have no issue stopping caffeine immediately while others take a few weeks. If you have been using your coffee pot as a cup, it may take longer. Coffee drinkers might find that a nice alternative is kava, Postum, Pero, Teeccino, Roma Kaffree, or Dandy Blend. You can find these at most health food stores or sections or you can order them online.

Substitutions for fruit includes low acid fruits such as pears, apricots, papaya and watermelon. For tea drinkers, non-citrus, herbal or other non-caffeinated tea blends are a great alternative. Although water is always the best beverage of choice, grape juice is a nice thirst quencher that is not as irritating to the bladder.

Cigarette smoking is also irritating to the bladder surface and is associated with bladder cancer. Also, the coughing associated with smoking may lead to increased stress incontinence episodes. If you smoke, consider cessation as quickly as possible.

Sandy's Story

Sandy was a 68-year-old woman who was referred to me for urinary urgency and frequency. She was urinating approximately every hour during the day and was getting up four to five times per night to urinate. She was understandably frustrated and exhausted. She also experienced stress urinary incontinence (SUI) when coughing and had scar tissue in her lower abdomen from two C-sections.

The first thing Sandy and I did was look over a three-day diary of what she was eating, drinking, and at what times per day she was urinating. She was drinking three cups of coffee per day, enjoyed spicy food several times per week, and was using a large wedge of lemon in her water bottle each day.

After educating Sandy in the common bladder irritants, her symptoms reduced significantly after two weeks. She decreased coffee consumption to one cup per day, stopped eating spicy foods, and began drinking her water plain. Her treatment continued for a few weeks while we worked on improving her pelvic floor strength and softened her scar tissue. The urgency was no longer an issue, so Sandy was almost ready to discontinue her pelvic physical therapy because she had met her goals.

On one of her last visits, she came in and told me that on a whim she had decided to indulge in some spicy Mexican food. Sandy noticed, that after weeks of no urgency symptoms and only getting up once per night, her symptoms of getting up at night four or five times returned for that one night following the spicy meal. She reported to me that she had been so pleased with her progress because she could see the distinct correlation between her urgency and what she ate.

And then I asked Sandy if the Mexican meal was worth it. She smiled coyly and said, "I won't make a habit of it, but that particular meal truly was." So, this case shows how when you control what you eat and monitor your body's response, you can control your bladder. Yes, it is okay to indulge once in a while if the meal is truly worth it to you.

Chapter 5

Pelvic Organ Prolapse: Why It Feels Like Your Organs are Falling Out of Your Body

Pelvic organ prolapse (POP) is a condition when one or more of your pelvic organs presses into the walls of your vagina. This usually occurs due to stretching or weakening of the pelvic floor muscles or their ligaments. Also, POP can happen after pregnancy and childbirth. Women may also develop POP from prolonged, heavy lifting or exercise.

Also, some chronic conditions such as obesity, constipation or prolonged periods of heavy coughing can cause POP. Although POP is not life-threatening, it can cause pain, fear and issues with the bladder or bowels. It can also lead to an overall decreased enjoyment in life. POP causes a sensation of pressure in the pelvis or vagina. This condition is due to an imbalance of pressure in the thorax and support in the pelvic floor muscles.

Often, you can feel the descended organs by placing a finger into the vaginal opening. They may also be viewed using a hand-held mirror to observe the vaginal opening. It may feel as though your pelvic organs have become heavy or they are falling out of your body. The feeling of pressure may be worse in the evening, or after exercise or physical exertion, such as heavy lifting.

It is common to experience odd dribbling after urination, especially when standing up from the toilet to pull up your underwear or zip your pants. It may be difficult to have a bowel movement, and you may feel the urge to push in the vagina to assist the bowel movement along. This maneuver is called splinting and is often harmless if you use gentle pressure by stroking the inside of the vagina outwards to coax the feces outward.

Women with POP often experience other symptoms of pelvic floor weakness, including urinary incontinence and anal incontinence (fecal or gas leakage). POP is sometimes due to the tearing and weakening of the pelvic floor muscles or to the ligaments suspending the organs. It is estimated that 50 percent of women who have had a child will experience prolapse to some extent. Age also is a factor, with 50 percent of women over the age of 50 developing POP.[1]

Prolonged pushing during labor and delivery, such as pushing for longer than two and a half hours, tearing of the pelvic floor during childbirth, and the delivery of a large baby are all factors that can lead to prolapse. Women who have more than one child are at a higher risk for POP to occur. Women who have undergone a C-section can also experience POP, especially if they pushed during labor before undergoing a C-section. Women with POP should avoid sit-ups, crunches and heavy lifting, as this can worsen the prolapse.

Healthcare professionals classify POP depending on which organ or organs have dropped into the pelvic bowl. The classifications are as follows:

- **Urethrocele**: A prolapse of the urethra through the lower anterior vaginal wall.

- **Cystocele**: A prolapse of the bladder through the upper anterior vaginal wall.

- **Uterovaginal**: A prolapse in the descent of the uterus, cervix and upper portion of the vagina.

- **Rectocele**: A prolapse of the rectum into the lower wall of the vagina

- **Enterocele**: A prolapse of the upper back part of the vagina involving parts of the small intestines.

A conservative treatment plan consists of pelvic floor strengthening for women with mild POP, especially those who are still in their childbearing years. Women who experience POP and wish to have more children can strengthen the pelvic floor before and during pregnancy to limit the progression of POP. In addition to the exercises listed in this chapter, it is important to adopt some good lifestyle habits.

Avoiding constipation is imperative, which we will discuss this in a later chapter. Sitting and standing with good upright posture will reduce the pressure over the abdomen, as well. Avoiding the Valsalva maneuver, or bearing down while lifting heavy items, children, or exercising is extremely important. Training the pelvic floor muscles to contract prior to and during lifting, coughing, and sneezing will help protect the pelvic floor and organs. It can even stop or slow the progression of POP.

Breathing Exercises to Help Your POP

Learning to breathe properly is an essential part of healing POP. Sometimes women with POP breathe shallowly and through their chest instead of evenly through the abdomen and sides of the rib cage. By learning to breathe through the belly and sides of the rib cage, it is possible to improve overall circulation and reduce the strain on the pelvic floor muscles. Also, it reduces tension in the neck, head and shoulders.

To breathe properly, practice the following exercises. It is often best to couple this training with pelvic floor muscle training. Here's how to start:

- Find a comfortable position lying down.

- It is helpful to put pillows or a bolster under the knees to reduce tension in your lower back.

- Place one hand on the sternum or breastplate bone, and the other on the stomach.

- The goal of this breathing exercise is to keep your chest still and allow your stomach to rise and fall with each breath.

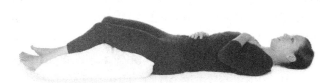

Next, follow these steps:

- Breathe in slowly and deeply through your nose.

- Allow your stomach to gently rise and keep your chest still.

- Exhale slowly and gently through your mouth, allowing your stomach to gently fall.

- Pay close attention to your stomach rising and falling as you breathe in through your nose and out through your mouth.

- Continue to take nice, slow breaths as you allow all thoughts and disruptions to fade away.

- Visualize the tension in your body being released.

Understanding the Role of Scar Tissue in POP

As discussed above, POP is a condition created when the pressure in your abdominal cavity is greater than the pelvic floor muscles can support. This leads to the dropping of the pelvic organs into the pelvic bowl. Scar tissue in the abdomen or pelvis can contribute to higher pressure in the abdomen. Surgical scars from an appendectomy, C-section, or even a laparoscopic procedure in the abdomen or pelvis can lead to restriction in your trunk.

The restriction from surgery can cause pressure on your uterus, bladder and bowl. Scar tissue is thick and stiff. However, it is possible to soften scars and create more pliability and mobility around them by utilizing gentle scar mobilization techniques. For some women, old scars can be painful and cause anxiety and fear whenever someone touches them. So, it is helpful to observe the scar in the mirror.

You can use a makeup brush to gently sweep along the scar to begin desensitizing it. This allows you to introduce gentle touch to the sensory receptors in the scar and surrounding tissue. Practice sweeping circles around the scar and brushing up and down and along the scar for five minutes per day. Do this until the makeup brush exercise is no longer painful or fear-inducing.

Here's how to mobilize a scar in your abdomen:

- Place your fingers directly on top of the scar.

- Apply the kind of pressure you would use to check a tomato for ripeness. It should be firm, but not so much that you squish the tomato.

- Apply this pressure and gently move your fingers upward and downward ever so slightly, inching your way along the length of the scar.

- Practice moving your fingers back and forth, as well.

- Next, gently pinch the skin immediately around the scar and pull it slightly away from your body, again moving the length of the scar.

- Repeat this practice daily for five minutes or so for three to four weeks.

Improving the mobility of your scar will help soften the tissue and decrease the restricted movement patterns and pressure that may contribute to POP. If the scars in your abdomen are significant, you have had multiple surgeries, or the scar tissue feels extra thick, see a physical therapist who specializes in pelvic health.

They are trained in scar tissue or visceral mobilization. So, a physical therapist can safely use manual techniques to soften your scars. Softening scars helps you restore the proper movement in your abdomen and pelvis. This will address your POP and pelvic pain symptoms.

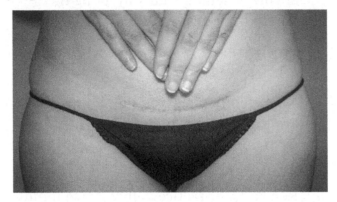

Place fingers just 1-2 finger widths above the scar for mobilization and then below for the first week or two. When you are feeling more comfortable, place fingers directly onto the scar for mobilization.

How to Fix Your POP

Moderate cases of POP are curable with specific pelvic floor strengthening exercises, such as Kegels. Kegels to address POP increase both the overall strength and endurance of the muscles. A long day at work, heavy walking, or physical exertion when lifting a child or going for a run, requires that you retrain your muscles to withstand that pressure.

Another Proven POP Exercise: Bottom on Pillows Kegels

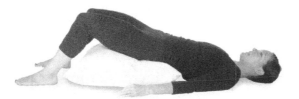

Here's how to do bottom on pillows Kegels:

- Lay down on the floor face up with two fluffy pillows under your hips.

- Bend your knees and plant your feet shoulder-width apart.

- Inhale and relax.

- Then exhale gently while you simultaneously contract your pelvic floor muscles. Imagine you are pulling a marble from the opening of the vagina up and into your vagina as far as possible.

- Try to hold for five seconds, and then inhale and relax the muscles.

- Repeat this exercise 10 times and do three or four sets each day.

As You Progress

As you get stronger, increase your pelvic floor strength by performing Kegels in these progressively more challenging positions:

- Remove the pillows and lie flat on your back with your knees bent and feet planted shoulder-width apart.

- In the seated position.

- While standing.

- Using the advanced exercises in Chapter 8.

It is beneficial to see a pelvic floor physical therapist for instructions on the safe progression of your POP exercises. Severe cases of POP may require a pessary device or surgery. A pessary is a device that helps support the organs in the pelvic bowl. They come in a variety of shapes and sizes. Your doctor or health care professional can prescribe and fit a pessary device for you.

It may require a trial period to get the best shape and style. Pessaries generally fit similarly to a contraceptive diaphragm or come in the shape of a ring like a baby's teething ring. You can remove some pessaries whenever you need for cleaning or sex and then insert it afterward. But some may need a healthcare practitioner to remove, clean and replace it.

Either way, you should be able to achieve a great fit that reduces your symptoms. The right pessary will enable you to exercise and do what you want in life without your POP symptoms. There are approximately 400,000 POP surgeries per year. However, POP surgery tends to have a 30 percent failure rate in the U.S. (DeLancey 2007). So, be sure to consider opting for surgery carefully.

Conservative treatments including pelvic floor strengthening, weight loss and activity modification are highly recommended prior to undergoing surgery for POP. There are several support groups both in person and online for women struggling with the emotional ramifications of POP. The Association for Pelvic Organ Prolapse Support (APOPS) is an excellent resource for women who seek support and other resources including healthcare providers specializing in POP.

Resources

1. Balmforth J. and Robinson D. "Pelvic Organ Prolapse." In *Pelvic Floor Dysfunction and Evidence Based Physical* Therapy, edited by Bo B., Bergmans B., Morkeed S., Van Kampen M., 233-248. Edinborough: Elselvier Publishers, 2007.

2. Delancey J. O. L., Morgan D. M., Fenner D. E., Kearney R., et al. "Comparison of Levator Ani Muscle Defects and Function In Women With and Without Pelvic Organ Prolapse." In *Obstet Gynecol* 109 (2007): 295-302.

Chapter 6

Kegels, Pelvic Floor and Core Strengthening

Pelvic floor and core strengthening are recommended for women who experience urinary and fecal incontinence, pelvic organ prolapse, issues with sexual response, hip, and lower back pain. A health care practitioner and a pelvic physical therapist should evaluate any woman who experiences chronic or ongoing pelvic pain before they engage in a pelvic floor or core strengthening program.

Importantly, while these exercises may address some forms of pelvic pain, they can also exacerbate a painful pelvic floor. In this chapter, you will learn what a Kegel is and how to incorporate Kegels into core stability exercises. You'll learn how to establish a well-rounded exercise program to address your pelvic weakness issues. There is also a section on Kegel devices for enhanced training.

What is a Kegel?

As you will remember from Chapter 2, a Kegel is the contraction of the pelvic floor muscles. The activation of the muscles, when you perform it properly, will create a pull of the muscles up and into the pelvic bowl.

How to Do a Basic Kegel

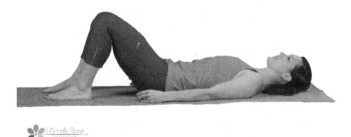

How to do a basic Kegel:

- First, inhale and relax all your muscles.

- Gently exhale as if you were cooling off hot food while simultaneously contracting your pelvic floor muscles as if you were shutting off the flow of urine.

- Hold the contraction for five seconds, then rest for five seconds.

- Repeat 10 times.

- Do three to four times every day until the rhythm becomes easy and almost second nature.

Here are some Kegel variations you can try:

- **Quick Kegels**: Quick Kegels are a method of pelvic floor training for stress urinary incontinence when coughing, sneezing or laughing. This contraction trains the muscles to respond quickly and strongly to rapid force. Here's how:

    o While seated, contract your pelvic floor muscles as quickly and as tightly as you can for one second.

    o Rest for five seconds and repeat 10 times.

    o Do this exercise three times every day.

- **Long Kegels**: When you can hold the basic Kegel for five seconds easily, begin to increase the hold time. Work toward a 10-second hold, followed by a 10-second rest. Perform 10 repetitions three times every day.

How to Prevent Leakage During High Exertional Activities

To train the pelvic floor muscles to react quickly and prevent urine leakage during higher exertional activities like exercising and lifting heavy objects, it is necessary to exercise them during such tasks. The goal of these exercises is to build coordination and control of the pelvic floor muscles during daily activities, such as walking, climbing stairs, running and grocery shopping. To do this, perform the following exercises three to five times per week:

The Bridge

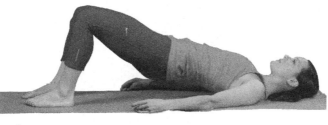

Here's how to do the bridge:

- Lie flat on the floor on your back with your hands at your side and your knees bent. Place your feet around shoulder width.

- Inhale and relax.

- Exhale and do a Kegel, and simultaneously lift your hips up off the ground.

- Continuing to exhale and maintaining a Kegel, slowly set your hips back down.

- Inhale and relax, then repeat 10 times.

Leg Lifts

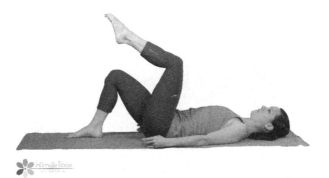

To do leg lifts, begin by lying down on your back with your knees bent and feet shoulder-width apart. Follow these steps next:

- Inhale and relax.

- Exhale and do a Kegel, and simultaneously lift one leg up as if you were marching, then slowly lower it down with control.

- Inhale and relax, then repeat the movement on the opposite side. Avoid holding your breath and remember to maintain the Kegel throughout the entire marching motion, both up and down.

- Perform 10 on each side.

Do the following exercises in the standing position. In the standing position, the pelvic floor is directly challenged because it has to work upright against gravity. These exercises are more challenging than seated Kegels because you perform them without the additional feedback of the seat to help the brain coordinate and contract the muscles. You can do these exercises using the regular Kegel contraction pattern or by using a vaginal weight. For safety, perform these exercises at the kitchen counter for additional balance when necessary.

The Standing Kegel

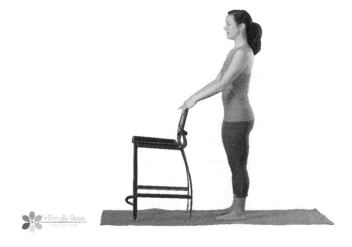

To do the Standing Kegel:

- Stand up tall with good posture, feet hip-width apart.

- Inhale and relax.

- Then exhale and simultaneously do a Kegel, holding the Kegel while exhaling for five seconds.

- Inhale and relax.

- Repeat 10 times.

The Standing Heel Raise Kegel

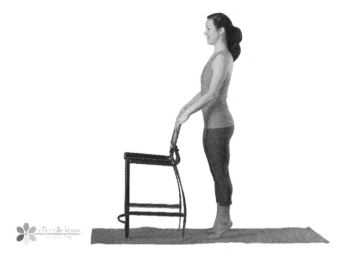

To do the Standing Heel Raise Kegel:

- Stand at your kitchen counter for support.

- Inhale and relax.

- As you exhale, simultaneously do a Kegel and slowly rise up and onto the balls of your feet, and then come back down with control.

- Once your feet are flat on the floor again, inhale and relax the pelvic floor, then exhale and repeat.

- You should feel the Kegel throughout the entire process of rising up and onto your toes and lowering them back down.

- Repeat 10 times.

The Mini Squat Kegel

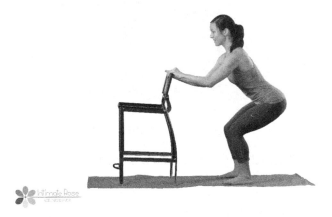

Follow these steps to do the Mini Squat Kegel:

- Stand at your kitchen counter for balance and support.

- Inhale and relax.

- Exhale and simultaneously do a Kegel, and then bend your knees to approximately 45 degrees while pressing your hips backward as if you were going to sit in a chair.

- Maintaining the Kegel, return to standing.

- Continue the Kegel and the gentle exhale throughout the entire duration of the movement.

- Once you return to standing, inhale and relax.

- Repeat 10 times.

Standing Side Kick

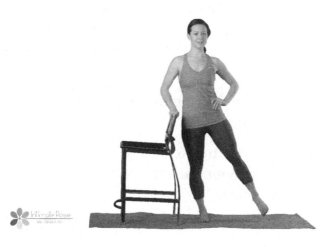

Here's how to do the Standing Side Kick:

- Stand with your feet together.

- Inhale and relax.

- Exhale and simultaneously do a Kegel, then slowly kick one leg out to the side and return it back to its starting place.

- Repeat 10 times.

All About Vaginal Weights

No, this section is not about lifting a surfboard with your pelvic floor muscles (yes, apparently that is a thing), although if you can do it, more power to you. There was mention of vaginal weights in Chapter 2; here we will discuss them in greater detail because they relate to further training your pelvic floor muscles.

Vaginal weights came along in the 1980s to help women retrain their weakened pelvic floor muscles. These weights help women strengthen their vaginal muscles through resistance. They also enable them to identify the correct muscles for performing Kegels. With vaginal weights, if you do a Kegel wrong, for example, by pushing down or holding your breath to bear down, the weight will fall out.

This notion of the brain's ability to identify and properly use a muscle is called proprioception. You can also use vaginal weights to perform the Kegel exercises in the basic and advanced Kegel exercises section.

How to Use Electronic Kegel Exercisers

There is a wide variety of electronic Kegel trainers currently on the market. They utilize an electronic sensor that you place into the vagina like a tampon. They also use a visual terminal of some sort. Some devices sync with a smartphone via an app. These apps provide basic visual feedback on the intensity and duration of the pelvic floor muscle contraction, such as a bright line that rises and falls as you perform Kegels.

Some apps show an icon on the screen that moves up and down along with pelvic floor muscle contractions. The app challenges you to utilize your muscles to push the icon upward and hold it for a given amount of time. There are fun competitions and advancement in levels as you become more skilled at performing Kegels. This provides motivation and is a great way to track progress.

Some units come with their own portable screens that attach to the vaginal sensors via wires. The visual screens range in complexity from simple lines rising and falling, to images of flowers opening and closing. However, electronic Kegel exercise programs tend to be expensive, ranging from $199 to $3,000 for a portable unit. Because they rely on technology, if something goes wrong with the unit, they are difficult to fix.

So, if the unit doesn't come with a warranty, you are left with nothing more than an expensive paperweight. Furthermore, the primary goal of an elcctronic Kegel exerciser is to provide feedback as to whether the user is doing their Kegel exercises properly. However, some devices are not sensitive enough to pick up on the slightest of contractions. So, the user is told that no contraction is happening when, in fact, the musclcs are beginning to work. They are simply not contracting to the level that the device can sense. Some units also have difficulty sensing muscle contractions when they are too close in proximity to other electronic devices. This even includes those that run on regular electricity, such as overhead lighting, microwaves, ceiling fans and televisions. In addition, vaginal weights can fill the primary role of the electronic Kegel exerciser if the user uses the wrong muscles.

For instance, when contracting the abdominals instead of the pelvic floor muscles, the weight pushes downward and out of the body. This informs the user immediately that they used the wrong muscles. In fact, they created vaginal weights with the goal to provide resistance to the pelvic floor muscles. Vaginal weights provide the instant feedback that lets the user know if they are using the muscles properly.

Importantly, if you have any hardware or devices in your body like an intrauterine device (IUD), metal or other materials from surgery (pins and screws), joint replacements, or a pacemaker, you can't safely use an electronic Kegel device. The electricity can interfere with cardiac pacemakers and may impact other devices.

So, if you want an easy, cost-effective way to strengthen your pelvic floor muscles to address bladder leakage or pelvic organ prolapse in a timely fashion and with the ability to multitask, then vaginal weights may be for you. They don't require you to sit and watch a screen. They don't require wires, batteries or chargers. They are discreet and easy to take with you when you travel. Plus, with a color-coding system like Intimate Rose's, they allow you to clearly track your progress by moving from one color up to the next.

For more information on how to do Kegels, how to use vaginal weights to reach your goals, visit *www.IntimateRose.com.*

Chapter 7

Constipation

Although many people joke about it, constipation can be one of the most uncomfortable of all the digestive issues. In fact, it is responsible for 13 million days of restricted activity and 2.5 million physician visits per year.[1] Constipation affects children, men, and women, though women and children experience it most commonly. However, it can be hard to treat because it has so many causes.

Some factors that lead to constipation include medications and hormonal changes. Things like diet and inactivity can lead to constipation, as well. Other issues include a restriction in or an incoordination of the pelvic floor muscles during the defecation process. However, more serious illnesses like colon cancer and anal fissures may be the cause of constipation. Therefore, it is a wise idea to visit your physician to discuss your constipation, especially if it is a relatively new issue.

Constipation: Is It Time for a Change?

When you need to plan your week around when you might possibly be able to have a bowel movement, you know it's time for a change. It is important to know what normal bowel movement patterns look like. On average, normal patterns of defecation are anywhere from three times per day to three times per week.[2]

There is a lot of variabilities, so if you are pooping two times per week without discomfort or issues emptying your bowel, that is normal for you. The bottom line is that going less frequently than three times per week is often considered constipation and is associated with discomfort and other health issues.

Also, the consistency of your poo is an indicator of how your body is processing the drinks and food you consume. Each trip to the bathroom tells the story of the previous few meals movements through your body. Keep in mind that in addition to what you eat, many factors affect how your body processes food and drink. Normal stool consistency is firm with lines in it, just like a Snickers bar (did I just ruin Snickers bars for you?).

The more firm it becomes, from a hard-looking sausage to something like rabbit pellets, the slower your digestive system is transitioning the food through your body. The softer and waterier your stool becomes, the faster your digestive system is processing food.

Women and Constipation

Women who experience constipation also commonly experience headaches, difficulty concentrating, depression, mood swings, a decline in energy, bloating, gassiness, and urinary issues. Urinary tract infections, leaking urine in bed at night, and urinary incontinence are all commonly associated with constipation.

It is important to check with your health care provider if you experience constipation to rule out diseases such as cancer and anorectal fissures. Your doctor can analyze your medications for drug-related causes. If you get a clean bill of health, it is helpful to know there are many non-surgical, natural measures that you can take to cure your constipation for good.

Medications that can cause constipation include, but are not limited, to the following:

- Antacids containing aluminum or calcium

- NSAIDs, such as ibuprofen and Advil

- Antiparkinsons drugs such as Sinemet or Levodopa

- Antidepressants

- Iron supplements

- Psychotropics

- Hypertension medications such as Clonidine, Lisinopril, Vasotec, and Capoten

- Diuretics

- Nasal decongestants and antihistamines

- Antispasmodics.

- Cholesterol medications

- Opiates such as Percocet, Percodan, Lortab, and Darvocet.

Other factors that can contribute to constipation include adhered scars in the abdomen or pelvic area. This includes scars from an appendectomy, as well as gallbladder and intestinal surgery. Procedures like hernia repair, cardiac stents and imaging scars in the groin can also cause constipation. Also, having a cesarean section, hystcrectomy, episiotomy or any surgery that leaves a scar between your collar bones and your knees can be problematic.

Scars can grow over and stick to the surface of the stomach, intestines, or rectum. However, the great news is, there are specialized mobilizations and massage techniques that can soften these scars and improve gut motility. Importantly, only licensed medical professionals, such as abdominal-pelvic floor physical therapists should perform such maneuvers.

Understanding the Common Types of Constipation

Did you know there are several types of constipation? Here is an overview of the most common types.

Functional Constipation: This type of constipation is due to transit issues in the colon or anus, where the feces comes out. It is characterized by difficulty passing stool most of the time, often for months or years consistently. Functional constipation may be due to your intestines not moving the stool through the system properly. Another cause is the difficulty of your anal sphincters pushing the stool out once it reaches the rectum or the end of the intestines.

However, you can relieve functional constipation by retraining the bowels in proper functioning and the anal muscles in how to propel the feces out of the body. A pelvic floor physical therapist trained in constipation and bowel issues can be of great help with this.

Pelvic Outlet Obstruction or Dyssynergic Defecation: This is a type of constipation that occurs because of issues between the anorectum and the pelvic floor muscles. This form of constipation affects 40 to 50 percent of people with constipation.[3] Common symptoms of a pelvic outlet obstruction or dyssynergic defecation include excessive straining to have a bowel movement and the feeling that you were not able to get it all out. Some women find that the only way to get fecal material out is by sweeping one or two fingers into the vagina to manually coax the feces out.

Women with this form of constipation commonly report urinary incontinence, frequency of urination or urgency, bladder pain, and pain with sex. They may also feel an aching sensation after sex, lower back pain, and pain in the inner thighs. Often, a lack of coordination of the pelvic floor muscles is a root cause of dyssynergic defecation. The treatment for this is a regiment of specialized exercise is biofeedback or the use of ultrasound imaging by a licensed and certified pelvic floor physical therapist.

Pelvic Organ Prolapse: This can also result in constipation. As we discussed in the POP chapter, it occurs when the organs in the pelvic bowl descend downward and press into the walls of the vagina. The vaginal wall is like a tent wall to the rectum. If there is pressure within that vaginal space from other organs, it can encroach on the rectum, making defecation difficult.

Rectal Prolapse: This is a condition in which the anal sphincter relaxes. It causes layers of the rectal wall to protrude through the opening and often outside of the anus. Often, people who have rectal prolapse experience a sense of pressure. Also, they can see or feel the layers of the rectal wall coming out of the anus after having a bowel movement. Women often experience this after years of straining to have bowel movements.

It can also happen after damaging the nerve to the sphincter from childbirth, pregnancy, or sometimes with natural aging processes. Contrary to management for POP, rectal prolapse often requires surgery. For women who are not surgical candidates or for more mild cases, pelvic floor strengthening and dietary changes are helpful in treating rectal prolapse.

How to Manage Most Forms of Constipation

The most important factor in the management of constipation is nutrition and diet. Eating 25 to 35 grams of fiber per day is important. Fiber increases the weight of your stool, so it speeds up colonic transport time.

Fiber also absorbs water extremely well, helping to produce softer, larger stools that the digestive system can pass more easily and quickly.[4] Foods that are high in fiber include fruits, vegetables, legumes, beans, and whole grains.

However, if you have food allergies or find it challenging to get enough natural fiber in your meals, supplementing them can help. Metamucil, Citrucel, and Fibercon are all fiber supplements that are easy to find at most grocery and drug stores, and even online.

Also, you should drink plenty of water, especially if you feel thirsty, and maintain daily physical activity for at least 30 minutes. Planning regular meal times is also helpful, especially breakfast. It is crucial to eat breakfast to initiate mobility in the colon after you have been lying in bed for several hours. You may also find that attempting to have a bowel movement within 20 to 30 minutes of eating is helpful, too. This is because eating produces the gastrocolic reflex. It is a reflex that causes the intestines to be more active during and immediately after eating.

Furthermore, when your body gives you the urge to defecate, you need to proceed to the restroom and go. Never hold it off. Studies show that people who have normal bowel movements and bowel patterns tend to empty their bowels at the same time each day.[5] This suggests that defecation is part of our body's conditioned reflex. Ritualized bowel habits and an established routine can aid in healthy bowels.

How to Create Your Constipation Diary

Start by keeping a diary for approximately seven days. In your diary, note at what time you eat meals and snacks as well as what time you tend to have bowel movements. Many people notice a trend in what time of day they generally have a bowel movement. Sometimes the trends show patterns of behavior, emotion, stress, or even scheduling issues.

For instance, I had a particular patient who worked part-time. She noticed after keeping a bowel diary that she did not have bowel movements on the days that she went into work. She also noted that her job caused her significant stress and anxiety. Recognizing these patterns allows you to make a shift in your daily schedule. Also, it may even reveal underlying issues that you may need to reconcile.

Why Positioning Matters

Positioning on the toilet is one of the easiest fixes for constipation. By using a Squatty Potty or other stool, you draw the knees up above the hips. This position places your pelvic floor in a mechanically relaxed and more open position to have a bowel movement. I wish I had a nickel for every patient case of constipation I helped cure just from teaching them the proper position and biomechanics.

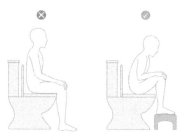

This image demonstrates proper toilet positioning with feet and knees elevated to relax and open the pelvic floor muscles for easier bowel movements.

Here's how to get the proper posture for more effective bowel movements:

- Push your clothing down below your knees so that they do not restrict motion at your hips or knees.

- Sit with your feet elevated on a Squatty Potty stool or yoga blocks so that your knees are higher than your hips.

- Bring your knees apart so that they are wider than your hips.

- Lean forward with a straight back and rest your elbows or hands on your knees.

- Use calm, quiet breaths to help relax the pelvic floor muscles.

- Press your belly out as if you were a Buddha, or like a bubble. Keep it pressed out and tighten the muscles to make it hard. Feel the drop of pressure into the pelvic floor.

- Push downward into the pelvic floor while gently exhaling as if you were blowing through a straw.

- Avoid straining or holding your breath at any point.

- Allow yourself to try for a bowel movement for five minutes on the toilet. If nothing happens, pull your pants up, move around using a variety of body movements, and try again in 20 to 40 minutes or when the urge becomes strong again.

If you find that you still need help addressing constipation, enemas and medications can help. I always encourage my patients to put effort into conservative methods such as diet, exercise, pelvic physical therapy, and proper mechanics before utilizing medications. However, in some cases, medications and further treatment are warranted.

Be sure to discuss your options with your physician. If you feel uncertain or uncomfortable with the recommendations, seek a second or even a third opinion to gather all the information possible, so you can make a good decision.

Emma's Story

Emma came to see me at the advisory of a general surgeon in town. She was 20 years old and had lived with constipation since she was able to remember. Her primary care physician sent her to a gastroenterologist, and the gastroenterologist recommended colon resection and referred her to a general surgeon due to the fact that she was unable to have bowel movements more frequently than once peer week. The recommended procedure would require the surgeon to cut into her abdomen and remove approximately 12 inches of colon. If this procedure failed, the surgeon would place a colostomy bag that would catch the feces through a portal in her abdomen. The general surgeon heard that I treat constipation and felt that a trial of pelvic physical therapy was warranted before removing a part of the colon of a 20-year-old woman.

After a lengthy discussion of her medical history and a thorough examination, I concluded that Emma had dyssynergic defecation. This meant she needed to learn the best positioning to have a bowel movement and we needed to teach her pelvic floor and sphincter muscles how to coordinate the motion of propelling the fecal material down and out of her body.

Emma's treatment consisted of a specific form of soft tissue massage in the abdomen and lower back to ensure that her muscles were not guarding or impinging the intestines. I educated her on the toileting mechanics earlier in this chapter. I also used what is called balloon-expulsion training to teach her body how to sense and propel fecal matter down and out, so that she could have proper bowel movements. Balloon expulsion involves using a special balloon connected to a catheter. The balloon is inserted into the rectum and filled with a precise amount of air to mimic fecal material. The patient is then guided to notice the sensation of the balloon filling, and then to properly co-ordinate their muscles to expel the balloon. This process trains the brain and the pelvic floor to have smooth, normal bowel movements.

After about two months of pelvic physical therapy, she was able to have regular bowel movements four times per week. Emma felt less pain and cramping in her stomach, too.

Most importantly, she knew that she would not have to endure surgery for colon resection. This is one of my favorite examples because she went through several different types of doctors and many years of pain and frustration before landing in my clinic.

Now Emma has proper bowel function after just two months of training. Remember, many forms of constipation are curable with only a few adjustments to your diet and proper muscle retraining. Just think of how you will use all that free time that you used to spend on the toilet waiting for something to happen!

Resources

1. Rao S. S. et al, "Dyssynergic Defecation: Demographics, Symptoms, Stool Patterns, and Quality of Life," *J Clin Ganstroenterol* 38 (2004): 680-596.

2. Walter S. A. et al. "Assessment of Normal Bowel Habits In the General Adult"

3. Rao S. S., "Treating Pelvic Floor Disorders of Defecation: Management or Cure?" *Curr Gastro Rep.* 11 (2009) :278-287.

4. Harris M. S., "Evaluation and Treatment of Constipation," *International Foundation for Functional Gastrointestinal Disorders* (2012).

5. Rao S. S., "Constipation: Evaluation and Treatment of Colonic and Anorectal Motility Disorders," *Gastroenterol Clin N Am.* 36 (2007) :687-711.

Chapter 8

Pelvic Pain

One chapter is never enough to dedicate to the topic of pelvic pain. If you are one of the one in seven women who experience pelvic pain, there is help available to you. The resources listed at the end of this chapter will help you get on your way to healing. There are entire clinics throughout the United States dedicated to treating pelvic pain with caring, compassionate clinicians who will listen and understand what you are saying.

You may have had every medical test, MRI, ultrasound, blood work, and colonic in the book and still wind up clean. A long string of physicians may have checked you over, shrugged their shoulders, and told you that you are fine. You may have been told to simply "relax", "have a glass of wine", "try lighting a candle", or other condescending statements about how to manage your pelvic pain. You may have racked up debt and tried many things yet still suffer in pain wondering what in the world is wrong with you. However, you are not crazy, nor is this "all in your head".

Pelvic pain often manifests in the soft tissue areas of the body that do not show up on medical tests. It is often a component of how your brain interprets signals from the pelvic organs and muscles. Pelvic pain often resolves when you address your trigger points or knots in the pelvic floor muscles, as well as scar tissue. Also, teaching coordination to the muscles in your pelvic floor can help, and recognizing when they are overactive. These are fixable and curable conditions, although they take time. Often some work with a talented and well-trained pelvic health professional is the key to unlocking pelvic pain.

Pelvic pain is a generalized term to describe a wide variety of diagnoses and conditions. It is often destructive in the lives of the men and women who experience it because the pelvis is a pertinent area of the body, in that you use it for the activities of daily living, your occupation and for recreation. Additionally, you use your pelvis for bowel and bladder function, sexual health and the list goes on and on. The pelvis is a component of everything you do and experience. Therefore, when it becomes a painful area of the body, it can be highly destructive. It is estimated that one in seven American women ages 18 to 50 experience pelvic pain. In fact, this condition accounts for 10 percent of gynecologic visits, 20 percent of laparoscopic surgery, and 12 to 16 percent of hysterectomies.[1]

Pain science has come a long way in many respects, but in some aspects, the medical field has failed to manage these diagnoses appropriately. The United States is currently experiencing an opioid crisis. The National Institute of Health (NIH) estimates that every day, more than 115 people die from an opioid overdose.[1] Yes that is right - every day.

Furthermore, pelvic pain is one of the more humiliating forms of pain because it interferes with both normal bodily functions, and the ability to engage in sex. Lack of intimacy can further drive feelings of despair, which can lead to substance abuse or other harmful behaviors, not to mention the decay of personal relationships.

There is so much to say on this topic. Many other pain scientists and physical therapists have created a movement to provide better education on this matter for people who are suffering from pelvic pain. Research shows that the more education you have on what pain actually is, what it means, and how to manage or cure it, the better off you are.[2] The definition of the broad term of chronic pelvic pain is having pain in the abdomen or pelvis that has lasted longer than three months. Also, it is not due to diseases such as cancer, endometriosis or dysmenorrhea.

Pelvic pain includes pain in the lower abdomen, vulva, vagina, perineum, anus, or tailbone. It is often accompanied by lower back pain and constipation in women. The common terms or diagnoses to describe some specific pelvic pain conditions include:

- Vaginismus
- Vulvodynia
- Vestibulodynia
- Coccydynia
- Dyspareunia

- Pain with Penetration

- Groin Pain

- Genital Pain

- Levator Ani Syndrome

- Pelvic Floor Tension Myalgia

- Non-Relaxing Pelvic Floor

- Pudendal Neuralgia

- Proctalgia Fugax

Treatment of chronic pelvic pain often begins with a thorough examination by a well-trained pelvic health physical therapist (PT). The pelvic PT will ask questions about your gynecological and other medical histories. Then they will take a close look at how your back, hips, and pelvis are functioning. The PT will assess scar tissue and will perform a brief vaginal examination to determine if you have trigger points, adhesions or scar tissue in your pelvic floor muscles.

They will analyze the pelvic muscle tone and how well the muscles can contract and relax. Often women who experience chronic pelvic pain have high tone in their pelvic muscles, meaning their muscles are active more than normal. Then the PT will then devise a plan to address your pain based on their findings. Treatments include gentle manual therapy to address trigger points in the pelvic floor, biofeedback to retrain the muscles in how to contract and relax on command, stretches and specific exercises.

This form of physical therapy is unlike other types of physical therapy in that it is highly specialized. Also, it is not a "no pain, no gain" form of treatment. A pelvic physical therapist is not going to ask you to perform exercises or movements that exacerbate your symptoms. Sometimes the muscles have become tight from chronic tension, gripping or holding patterns. This is often found in women who have experienced physical or sexual trauma.

Approximately 50 percent of women who have chronic pain have experienced sexual abuse at some point. This can range from an abusive childhood to a singular traumatic event or sexual trauma of any degree. If you have ever watched a dog put its tail between its legs in fear, you have witnessed a reflexive pelvic floor contraction. This tail between the legs maneuver is created via a contraction of the pelvic floor of a dog to protect itself and its reproductive organs. This behavior has been observed in human females when they are in a stressful or traumatic situation. Sexual abuse is also correlated with headaches, gynecological and gastrointestinal disorders, anxiety and panic disorders. Other traumatic events may also result in chronic pelvic pain. Birth trauma, illness, surgery, psychological abuse, the death of a loved one, natural disasters, and near-death experiences can all trigger chronic pelvic pain episodes. The brain and the body are closely connected, and not only to each other, but also to our essence as people.

When we are threatened or our lives are in danger, the rippling effects of vigilance to our bodies can remain for years, or even decades. Our brain has one job: to keep us alive and it may utilize this clenching or gripping of muscles in an attempt to subconsciously protect us. For this reason, it is also highly beneficial to seek counseling or therapy to address your underlying stress. Interestingly, "talk therapy" is often not beneficial.

In fact, many women find that the rehashing of the details of their trauma is harmful instead of helpful. However, seeking a counselor with a certification in sexual trauma, abuse, or a therapist who has trained in cognitive behavioral therapy (CBT) can be helpful. These therapists use different methods to change behaviors and belief systems, often without having their patient rehash a traumatic event.

Painful Bladder Syndrome and Interstitial Cystitis

Painful bladder syndrome is an umbrella term for pain in and around the bladder. It includes the medical diagnosis, Interstitial Cystitis or IC. To confirm IC, they use cystometry and urological testing to determine the presence of ulcerations inside the bladder walls. Women with IC often experience urinary urgency and pain with a full bladder. The good news is, you can reduce the symptoms of IC with dietary changes, manual therapy by a pelvic physical therapist, and modifications to daily routines. There are many great resources available including the book, *The Interstitial Cystitis Solution*[4].

Vaginismus

Vaginismus is vaginal tightness or muscle spasms that cause pain, burning, cramping, spasms, and difficulty or the inability to receive vaginal penetration. Women who experience vaginismus may also experience fear, general anxiety and the avoidance of certain activities including sex, as well as protective behaviors. These protective behaviors may include muscular guarding or clenching of the muscles in the pelvic floor, buttocks, hips, thighs, neck, chest and shoulders.

Women with vaginismus do not intentionally tighten or restrict their muscles. Rather, it is a reflexive response. This makes penetration difficult or impossible. When intercourse is attempted, it can feel like a partner is crashing into a brick wall. This causes extreme pain, frustration, and sadness for both partners.

Friction within the relationship is commonly experienced in couples with this issue. Various forms of counseling and sex therapy are extremely helpful. While health care providers may do certain tests and procedures, such as ultrasounds or lab testing to rule out disease, these tests will come back negative in women with vaginismus. However, once vaginismus is the diagnosis, there are gentle and non-invasive treatment methods that are helpful in overcoming the symptoms.

Some treatment options include pelvic physical therapy with a highly trained pelvic physical therapist and vaginal dilator training. This is worth repeating: counseling with a sexual health therapist or couples counselor is helpful in many instances. Participating in the physical and mental aspects of training while simultaneously receiving support from a counselor or therapist can teach couples new skills to support each other.

Often, a male partner simply does not know how to best support his female partner when vaginismus is involved. That can lead to further distress for both partners.

Vaginal Dilators As A Tool For Successful Vaginal Training for Vaginismus, Vestibulodynia, Vulvodynia, Pelvic and Vaginal Pain

Vaginismus and other vaginal pain treatments include the use of vaginal dilators while learning to relax the pelvic floor muscles. To decrease pain with vaginal penetration, the keys to success are consistency and routine practice. The daily use of vaginismus dilators, coupled with relaxation techniques and focused attention on training the muscles will result in achieving your goals.

Your health care provider may have a unique training plan for you outside of the recommendations made here. Therefore, always consult with a health care provider before starting a new training plan. Vaginal dilator therapy is beneficial for the following issues:

- Pain with Sex

- Vaginismus

- Vaginal Stenosis

- Vulvodynia

- Vaginitis

- Changes with Menopause

- Chronic Pelvic Pain

- Sjogren's Syndrome

- Androgen Insensitivity Syndrome (AIS) or MRKH

- Lichen's Sclerosis

- Gender Affirming Surgery

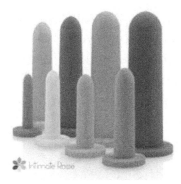

Vaginal dilators range in size, allowing for the progressive training of the pelvic floor muscles.

Gentle Yoga Poses for Vaginismus and General Pelvic Pain

Basic stretches can help alleviate some pelvic pain symptoms. Choose those that work for you and implement them as part of your daily routine.

The Happy Baby Stretch

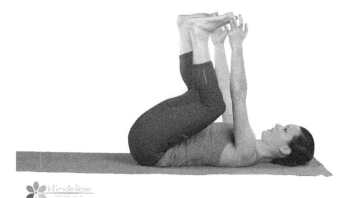

Follow these steps to do the Happy Baby Stretch:

- Lying on your back, bend you knees and bring your feet upward so that they face the ceiling.

- Grasp your toes if you can, or simply embrace the backs of your knees.

- Breathe deeply into the sides of the rib cage and through the belly.

- Hold this position for one to three minutes and then gently release.

Child's Pose Stretch

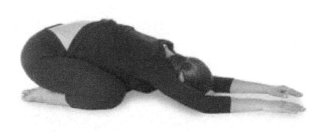

Follow these steps to do the Child's Pose stretch

- Kneeling, bring your knees wider than your hips

- Bring your arms parallel to your ears
- Breathe deeply into the sides of your rib cage and lower back

A variation: Pillow Behind the knees:

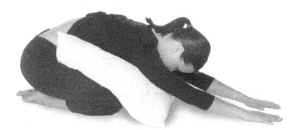

- Place a pillow behind your knees to bring a gentle opening stretch around the tailbone and posterior pelvic floor

- Gently breath into the lower back and expand the rib cage to the sides

- Relax the pelvic floor allowing it to gently release

A variation: Pillow In Hip Crease

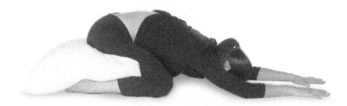

- Place a pillow in the crease of your hips
- Gently breath into the low back and pelvic floor
- Relax the pelvic floor allowing it to gently release

Deep Squat Stretch

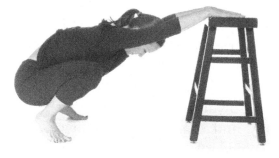

Deep Squat Head Down for a complete spine and pelvic stretch

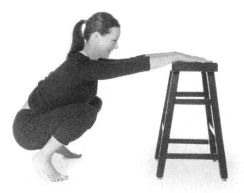

Deep Squat Head Up for a pelvic stretch more centered around the pelvic floor

Stacie's Story

Stacy was a 22-year-old patient who was referred to me by her women's health nurse practitioner. Stacie was newlywed and had been experiencing unbearable pain when trying to have sex with her new husband. Stacie did not have a history of sexual abuse, however, when growing up, her mother had been verbally and emotionally abusive. Thankfully she married a kind and patient young man and was in a safe relationship.

Stacie's greatest challenge was that she was new to sex. Every time sex her husband tried to initiate sex, her pelvic floor muscles would clench tightly, preventing penetration and making for a painful experience. Stacie was concerned her new husband's patience might run out if she was unable to fulfill him sexually.

Our treatment began by educating Stacie about pelvic floor anatomy and how the pelvic floor muscles can respond to uncertain situations by contracting and closing. Drawing awareness to how her muscles were behaving helped reduce Stacie's fear and anxiety tremendously. In the clinic, I utilized biofeedback so Stacie could learn to coordinate the relaxation and opening maneuver at the vaginal opening.

Also, I taught her the role of breathing in reducing the muscle clenching response, as well as how to prepare for sex by taking her time. Stacie learned how to control her muscles spasms by practicing at home with vaginal dilators, beginning with a small dilator and progressing to a larger one more closely resembling her husband. After three months of treatment, Stacie was able to engage in pain-free sex. She was ecstatic to learn that it could actually be enjoyable.

But Stacie was lucky to receive treatment at such a young age. I often receive female patients in their 50's and 60's who have gritted their teeth through pelvic pain for decades. If you are experiencing pelvic pain, please know that it is fixable, and you don't have to suffer. The next chapter will discuss breathing and how controlling your breath can be an effective tool in managing pelvic floor disorders of all types, especially pain.

Additional Reading on Pelvic Pain

- Why Pelvic Pain Hurts: Neuroscience Education for Patients with Pelvic Pain by Adriaan Louw, Sandra Hilton, and Carolyn Vandyken.

- Healing Pelvic Pain by Amy Stein.

- Pelvic Pain Explained: What You Need to Know by Stephanie Prendergast and Elizabeth H Akincilar.

- The Interstitial Cystitis Solution by Cozean, N, Cozean J.

- Meet Me: A JOURNEY THROUGH PELVIC PAIN (2018) by Amy Watkins.

Resources and Support for Pelvic Pain

International Pelvic Pain Society: https://pelvicpain.org/

Citations:

1. "Opioid Overdose Crisis," National Institute on Drug Abuse, last modified March 2018, https://www.drugabuse.gov/drugs-abuse/opioids/opioid-overdose-crisis.

2. Adriaan Louw, Sandra Hilton, and Carolyn Vandyken, *Why Pelvic Pain Hurts: Neuroscience Education for Patients with Pelvic Pain* (International Spine and Pain Institute, 2014).

3. Chronic Pelvic Pain (2014). Available at: https://bestpractice.bmj.com/topics/en-us/722

Chapter 9

The Importance of Breathing

Breathing seems like such an easy, automatic part of life. If you are alive, it is because your lungs are taking in and expelling air. Interestingly, there are efficient and inefficient ways of breathing that can affect your overall health and reinforce poor neuromuscular patterns. Often when there is pain in your body, your breathing becomes shallow and strained. Also, breath holding is common yet not conducive to good health.

Learning to breathe properly is an important part of healing pelvic floor muscle dysfunction as well as pelvic and vaginal pain. Many women with pelvic pain breathe shallowly and into their chests. By learning to breathe evenly through your belly, it is possible to improve overall circulation, reduce the strain on your pelvic floor muscles, and reduce tension in your neck, head, and shoulders.

How to Breathe Properly

To breathe properly, practice the following exercises. It is often best to couple this training with vaginal training if you experience pelvic or vaginal pain, which was discussed in Chapter 8. To start, find a comfortable position lying down. Often, it is helpful to put pillows or a bolster under your knees to reduce the tension in your lower back. Place one hand on your chest bone and the other on your stomach. The goal during this breathing exercise is to keep your chest still and allow your stomach to rise and fall with each breath.

How to Practice Diaphragmatic or Belly Breathing

- Breathe in slowly and deeply through your nose, allowing your stomach to gently rise while keeping your chest still.

- Exhale gently through your mouth as if you were blowing out birthday candles, allowing your stomach to gently fall.

- Pay close attention to your stomach rising and falling as you breathe in through your nose and out through your mouth.

- Continue to take slow breaths as you allow all thoughts and disruptions to fade away. Visualize the tension in your body being released as your body relaxes.

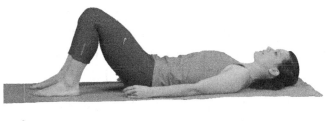

Body Scanning for Body Awareness

Body scanning is a helpful technique to couple your breathing practice with mind-body awareness. Mind-body awareness is an effective cornerstone of managing your pain, muscle weakness, tension, and incoordination. It is a technique that trains your brain and muscles to communicate better. Also, it allows you to become more aware of your own particular movement patterns and postures.

Throughout the body scan, you will be bringing awareness to how your body is positioned and how it feels in relation to the ground. The purpose of this exercise is to simply bring awareness of posture. The pressure that you experience in your joints, skin and various body parts gives your brain information that you may not have otherwise realized. By performing the scan while lying down, you can relax without fatiguing your muscles as you analyze each area of your body.

Resist the temptation to judge yourself or your body based on what you experience. This is simply a data-gathering exercise. Also, how you feel during your scan in the morning can be different from what you experience at night. Furthermore, the scan may feel different one day compared to the next. You may also begin to notice patterns of posture or muscular holding patterns. This allows you to have a deeper understanding of why certain areas of your body may feel sore, fatigued, tight or painful. By resisting judgement of yourself, you allow your brain to learn from the posture so you can change these patterns.

How to do a body scan:

Lie flat on your back in a comfortable space, with no pillows or bolsters under your legs, if you can tolerate it. The scan takes approximately 10 minutes, so if you have difficulty tolerating lying flat, you can use a small bolster pillow under your legs. However, you will gain the most beneficial information if you are lying flat.

- **Begin to breathe through your belly.** Take gentle breaths in through your nose, allowing your abdomen to rise. Breathe gently and slowly out through the mouth. Maintain this breathing pattern and bring your attention to your heels.

- **Ask yourself if your heels are experiencing equal pressure with the ground.** Does one heel feel heavier than the other? Does one feel like it's making more contact with the ground?

Is one rolled outward more than the other?

- **Move your attention upward to the relationship between the ground and the back of your knees**. Does the back of one knee feel flatter, or as though it is making more contact with the ground than the other? Does one knee feel more rolled out to the side? Do they feel equal?

- **Bring your attention to your gluteal muscles and your pelvis**. Does one side feel heavier than the other? Is one side in more contact with the ground?

- **Switch your attention up to your shoulder blades**. Does one shoulder blade feel as though it is closer to your ear than the other? Are they symmetric in height, or is one slid upward? Does one feel heavier?

- **Lastly, draw your attention to your head**. Ask yourself if your nose is tilted upward toward the wall behind you or downward toward the wall in front of you. Is your chin pressing toward your chest? Is your jaw tight and clenched? Are your brows furrowed? Are your eyes tightly closed?

- **Once you have completed the scan, note any patterns**. Did one leg feel heavier in each area? Did heavier body parts seem to relax after you noticed them clenching or compressing?

- **Next, perform the gentle pelvic clock exercise**. After completing the pelvic clock exercise, repeat the body scan, analyzing differences. The purpose of the pelvic clock exercise is to systematically contract and relax your muscles in your pelvis and abdomen.

How to Do the Pelvic Clock Exercise

The pelvic clock exercise is useful for training your pelvic floor, lower back, gluteal muscles, abdominals, and joint receptors. This exercise provides better coordination, control, and pain-free mobility. Ultimately, the pelvic clock exercise trains your muscles to listen to the commands your brain sends. It gives more accurate information back to your brain about the position and movements of your pelvis and lower back. The process, called proprioception, helps to decrease your pain and improve the overall fluidity of your movements.

To do the pelvic clock exercise, use the following steps (note to see the slight nuances in the pelvic position look closely at the angle of my hands on my pelvis):

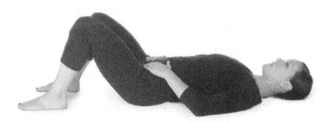

- Breathe using the diaphragmatic breathing pattern described above.

- When you inhale, notice a slight drop in your pelvis. This subtle pressure downward is a product of your diaphragm pulling downward into your abdominal cavity. The gentle force is transmitted through your body and down into your pelvic floor.

- When you exhale, notice that the pressure lifts as your diaphragm assists your lungs in expelling air.

Adding the 12-6 Pelvic Rock

The next step is to do the pelvic rock.

Imagine that your pelvis has a clock lying on top of it. The clock is arranged so that 12 o'clock is pointing toward your belly button and six o'clock is pointing toward your pubic bone. The hours three and nine are pointing toward the bony part of your pelvis on the left and right, respectively.

- **On the next inhale, notice that your pelvis rocks downward slightly toward the ground**. You will feel your tailbone come into contact with the ground. On the exhale notice how your pelvis rocks slightly and your tailbone comes up and away from the ground.

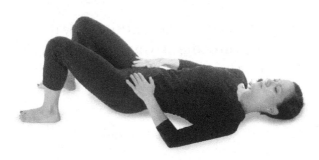

Pubic bone downward at 6'o clock- slight arch in back as pelvis tips downward

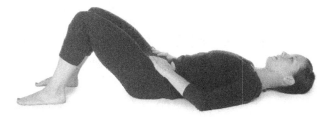

Pubic bone upward at 12 o'clock

- **Feel this gentle rocking of the pelvis with the pubic bone down in the six o'clock direction**, then rocking back up toward 12 o'clock. While keeping in mind that these movements are meant to be pain-free, small range, and controlled, begin to make the motion of rocking back and forth between 12 and six gradually larger.

- **If either position becomes painful, decrease the amplitude of the motion, making it smaller in range**. Repeat this gentle mobility exercise for one to two minutes. If you feel like your body could benefit from more, continue. If you feel that your pelvis is moving symmetrically and evenly from 12 to six, then move forward to the 3–9 pelvic rock.

- **Return the pelvis back to a comfortable position**. Continue to breathe through the diaphragm.

- **Expanding the Pelvic Rock to 3-9**

- **Visualize the clock on your pelvis again**. Imagine three o'clock and nine o'clock are overlying the bony protuberances on the front of your pelvis or the anterior superior iliac spine (ASIS), in fancy medical terminology.

- **Continue to gently breathe in through your nose and out through your mouth**. On the inhale, place pressure in your right heel and dip into three o'clock, or your left ASIS, pressing it toward the floor. You will feel a slight rotation in your pelvis, and your left knee will dip down slightly.

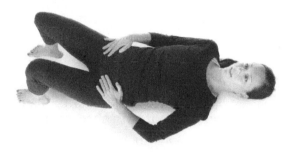

Left ASIS down 3 o'clock

- **Exhale and bring the three o'clock back up so that it is level with the rest of the clock.** Inhale and repeat this on your right side at nine o'clock by putting pressure into your left heel to sink your right ASIS downward.

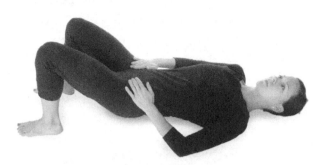

- **Exhale and bring it back up to level**. Repeat this process and take notice: Do your right and left sides move evenly? Does one side feel more challenging to move? If the answer is yes to the latter, gently seek symmetry. If the left is moving further than the right, see if the right can imitate its mate. Keep in mind that this motion should be gentle, pain free, and under control. Resist the urge to move quickly and resist the urge to push into pain.

- **Continue this process until both sides are moving equally or you have had enough.** A few minutes of practice is generally ample. However, if you are struggling, try to stay with the exercise until you feel a rhythm set in comfortably.

Move forward to the full clock, if you can. However, it may take a few days or weeks of practice of the 12-6 pelvic rock and 3-9 pelvic rock before you have the full control to move forward, and that is fine. Just be sure to move at your own pace.

How to Do the Full Pelvic Rock

- **While still lying on your back, visualize the clock on your pelvis again**. The movement you will complete is a circle of your pelvis in the clockwise direction, similar to a hula motion.

- **Inhale and rock your pelvis back toward 12 o'clock**. Do this while lifting your tailbone gently and slightly away from the ground.

- **From there, exhale and circle your hips toward three o'clock**. Use your abdominals, glutes, and pressure into your right foot to press your left hip into the ground.

- **Inhale and continue the circle**. Round into six o'clock with a slight pressure of your tailbone toward the ground.

- **Exhale and continue to nine o'clock**. Place some pressure into your left heel and use your abdominals to create a fluid and slow sweeping motion.

- **Inhale and continue the circle**. Go back up to 12 o'clock for a complete pelvic clock circle.

- **Continue for a moment or two and then reverse the motion to do it counterclockwise**. Analyze if one direction is easier for you than the other. If there is pain with any component of the exercise, remember, you are in control. You can decrease the range of motion and the speed to be in control for a pain-free experience.

- **After practicing the pelvic clock exercise, repeat the body scan**.

Analyze the symmetry in pressure beneath each section of your body. Ask yourself if they feel like each other. Analyze whether they feel different after the pelvic clock exercise. Often after practicing the pelvic clock, there is improved circulation through your legs, pelvis and low back.

Also, due to the rhythmic contracting and relaxing of the muscles within your pelvic floor and supporting muscles of your core and hips, you will experience decreased tension. Less tension will result in less pain and more comfort. This exercise is an easy-to-do practice and an instant crowd pleaser in my clinic.

After a few months of practicing the body scan lying down, consider repeating the body scan while standing, as well. The posture and holding patterns you utilize while standing will most likely feel completely different from those you feel while lying down.

Contract-Relax Tension Release Exercise

Another breathing technique enhanced by mind-body attention is the contract-relax tension release exercise. Practice releasing tension in your body, specifically in your pelvic floor muscles. Here's how:

- **Begin by focusing on your feet**. Your feet share common nerve roots with your pelvic floor, so it is helpful to practice noticing the muscles in your feet as they clench and unclench. Maintain your breathing pattern and clench your toes on both feet as hard as you can, making a "fist" with your feet for about five seconds.

- **Next, let your feet completely relax**. Then, clench them only halfway by giving a 50 percent effort toward clenching your feet for five seconds.

- **Again, allow your muscles to completely relax**. Notice how different they feel relaxed compared to clenched.

- **Do the same thing with your gluteal muscles or buttocks.** Maintain your breathing and don't hold your breath. Clench them together as hard as you can for five seconds, then relax. Do it again with a 50 percent effort for five seconds, then relax. Take note of the difference in sensation to clenched versus relaxed.

- **Now, do this with the pelvic floor muscles**. Contract them as hard as you can as if you were shutting off the flow of urine, then relax. Be sure to note the sensation of relaxation after they have clenched. Now perform a 50 percent effort contraction. Take note of the difference in the effort between clenching and relaxing.

- **Bring your attention to your abdominal muscles**. Keep breathing and contract these muscles as hard as you can by pulling your belly button in toward your spine. Hold for five seconds, then relax. Repeat this contraction at 50 percent effort, pulling your belly downward, and holding for five seconds, and then relax. As you relax, notice what it feels like to allow

your muscles to be still compared with
how they felt when they were clenched.

- **Finally, notice the tension around
  the shoulders, neck, and jaw**.
  Maintain your breathing, press your
  head slowly back into the pillow, and lift
  your shoulders toward your ears. Hold
  this for five seconds, then relax.
  Contract those muscles again, only this
  time at 50 percent of your strongest
  effort, and hold for five seconds, then
  relax.

Notice the sensation of your muscles when
they are fully relaxed. Continue breathing
deeply into your belly for a few more minutes
to conclude your practice. This exercise of
clenching, unclenching, and noticing the
sensation of relaxation is important because it
gives your brain information. This information
allows you to be more aware of clenching
patterns that may arise throughout your day
during times of stress, anxiety or pain.

Having the ability to clench and unclench
your muscles and breathe allows you to, little
by little, decrease the clenching pattern over

time. The goal is that if your muscles begin to clench, your brain will notice immediately because it has learned to monitor this pattern. Then it will automatically relax your muscles.

These exercises should help you become more aware of how your body works. You'll be able to release the tension in your muscles, which will lead to less pain and soreness. Be patient and take your time to master each exercise before moving on to the next.

Chapter 10

To Infinity and Beyond

Women's bodies are miraculous. The intricacy of balance in hormones, the orchestra of anatomical organs, and the sheer phenomenon of conceiving and growing another human are only the most apparent examples of this. For generations, women have endured and thrived through some of the most extenuating of circumstances.

Consider what it may have been like for a pioneer woman to travel the Oregon Trail using grass to catch menstrual blood under layers upon layers of underclothing. Imagine wearing those long, heavy dresses in the heat, snow, and, according to the infamous Apple Macintosh video game, apparently cholera and snake bites, too.

If your lady parts are painful, leaking, withholding, or prohibiting you from being all you are meant to be, I urge you to seek help from an experienced health care provider. If you don't currently have a provider who listens to you, it is time to switch. Patronizing health care is leading to underdiagnosing of diseases in women. The issues we discussed in this book are curable, although they take time and the right health care provider, including a well-trained pelvic physical therapist.

Diagnoses such as pelvic pain, constipation, and interstitial cystitis may feel oppressive and daunting. They often require having a few different care providers on board to manage the symptoms, but these people are out there. You may have had 19 surgeries and feel as though you have turned over every rock. But please keep looking. There are resources listed throughout this book to help you on your way.

I'll close this book with one final patient story. Interestingly, this patient belonged to my husband who is in the field of cardiology, although this is most certainly a pelvic story if ever I've heard one. The patient was a 76-year-old woman who was having an echocardiogram image done of her heart in the cardiac catheterization lab. The imaging procedure involves weaving a wire from the artery in her groin all the way up and into her heart. The preparation for the procedure involves shaving the groin and using antiseptic to prevent infection.

My husband greeted the patient and explained the procedure. He told her, "Ma'am, I'm going to have to lift your gown and remove your underwear to prepare for this procedure. Is that okay?" Without missing a beat this sharp woman told him, "Oh, I don't wear underwear, honey. My husband wants me ready at all times."

This story makes me laugh for so many reasons. She was unapologetic in her sexuality and her willing participation in it. At first glance, it may sound patronizing that a woman put herself at her husband's beck and call and ready for sex at any moment. However, my husband reports that her tone wasn't subservient. It was matter-of-fact and she had a little glimmer in her eye.

This woman reminds me that societal expectations are often untrue. You can have sex at any age if you choose to - or not. You can mend your body after delivering babies, after trauma or abuse, after constipation and after cancer. As a woman, you are resilient. But your body needs you to listen and take active participation in the healing process. Showing up and doing the work daily is necessary, and it works.

Resources:

To find a pelvic physical therapist:

1. American Physical Therapy Association's Section on Women's Health Pelvic Physical Therapist Locator: *http://pt.womenshealthapta.org/*

2. Herman and Wallace Pelvic Institute Pelvic Practitioner Locator: *https://pelvicrehab.com/*

3. Intimate Rose Solutions for Women's Health: *www.IntimateRose.com*

4. Educational Resources in several languages available at My Pelvic Floor Muscles: *www.Mypfm.com*

Acknowledgements

I am in deep gratitude to all the people that I work with. To Aaron Wilt for helping to make this book a reality. Behind every dream I have had for women's health initiatives in the past 3 years he has been behind them making things happen. To Micheala Begg for her always beautiful photos and patience with me in my new ventures. To the pelvic PT's who have trail blazed a new way of health care delivery, including those who have taught me in the APTA Section on Women's Health. To Patricia Koehler for fixing me and starting me on my new path. To my parents for demonstrating hard work and service to others. Not least, to the three men who live in my home for being patient with me while I take care of other people, write a book, do research, and teach students. To the two little ones for being sweet and adorable and to my husband for urging me to share my stories and experiences to promote women's health. A million thanks.

Made in the USA
Las Vegas, NV
08 March 2021

19199447R00089